TINNITUS

TAKE CONTROL

(TREATMENTS FOR TINNITUS RELIEF)

CHRIS SCIRE

PUBLISHERS INFORMATION

Copyright © 2014 Chris Scire

This edition published in 2014 by Kindle Publishing Pathway

ISBN-13:978-1499280722

ISBN-10:1499280726

WHY I WROTE THIS BOOK

I wrote this book because of the many patients who come to my clinic who have been told just "to live with their tinnitus" or just "to get on with it".

They were never told that there are many different strategies and techniques that could help them with managing their tinnitus.

I was really surprised when researching for this book that very little was written about the best treatment for tinnitus. Everyone who has ever suffered from tinnitus needs to know about this.

Why You Should Read This Book

This book will help you to realize that you do not have to put up with tinnitus and its effects, allowing it to dominate your life.

You can take control of your tinnitus by putting into action the strategies that I am going to share with you in this guide.

I also reveal the little known, proven best method for the treatment of tinnitus

The message of this book is that there is hope for the tinnitus sufferer. It is time for you to take control of your tinnitus.

TABLE OF CONTENTS

Chapter 1. What Is Tinnitus?

Before we begin to look at taking control of your tinnitus, it is useful to gain an understanding of just exactly what is tinnitus.

A Definition Of Tinnitus

The medical term tinnitus takes its origin from the Latin word for 'ringing'. Tinnitus can best be defined as the conscious experience of noise or noises but with no apparent external source.

Some people think that it is a disease or illness but in fact it is a symptom that has been generated from within the auditory system. Generally, tinnitus is only heard by the person who is experiencing it.

The Nature Of Tinnitus

The nature and intensity of tinnitus varies greatly from person to person. People report a variety of sounds such as buzzing,, hissing,whistling, roaring, clicking and of course ringing in their ears. People have even reported that their tinnitus sounds like music.

Most people only really become aware of their tinnitus at night when it is quiet. Some others find tinnitus to be too loud and disruptive, whilst other people have tinnitus that beats in time with their pulse. There are some people that even have a combination of different sounds. The tinnitus can be experienced as continuous, intermittent or transient.

Chapter 2. Who Gets Tinnitus?

Tinnitus can be experienced by all age groups. It does not discriminate at all. Some people experience it on a temporary basis whilst others have tinnitus permanently.

Some Demographics

It is generally considered that approximately 15% of world population has tinnitus. With 80% of tinnitus patients have some evidence of accompanied hearing loss. With only 10- 25% of tinnitus sufferers seeking medical attention.

Some Facts About Tinnitus In The UK

About 10% of adults, or six million people, have constant mild tinnitus. Up to 1% of adults ,approximately 600,000 people have tinnitus that affects their quality of life. Up to 30% of over 70s experience tinnitus, compared to 12% of people in their 60s and just 1% of people aged under 45. (Source: Action on Hearing Loss Information, July 2011)

SOME FACTS ABOUT TINNITUS IN THE US

About 10 percent of adults in the United States have experienced temporary tinnitus lasting at least five minutes. This amounts to nearly 24 million Americans. (Source: NIDCD)

Chapter 3. What Causes Tinnitus?

The actual causes of tinnitus are still not fully understood. Some maintain that the origin is somewhere within the auditory nerve while other theories assume that tinnitus can occur from damage anywhere in the auditory system. What is known is that tinnitus is associated as a symptom with a number of factors.

Hearing Loss

As people age and "wear and tear" takes place, the delicate hair cells of the inner ear reduce in number. It is this gradual change that causes an age related hearing loss (presbycusis). The overall effect of this is a reduction in the number of electrical signals being received by the brain. The latest research has shown that this lack of analysis can make the neurons in the brain more sensitive to sound due to them having to search for the signals that are no longer being sent by the ear. In effect, they become hyperactive. It is this hyperactivity that makes the brain receptive to the electrical noise of the neurons which it perceives as tinnitus.

Exposure To Loud Noise

There is sufficient evidence to show that people who work in loud noisy environments are at risk of developing tinnitus. This includes working with guns, power tools, road drills, involvement with explosions, various genres of music, factory machinery and even in night clubs. Put simply, a noise induced hearing loss is the result of a sound being loud enough for long enough, to cause damage the sensitive hair cells of the inner ear, either through exhaustion or by obliteration of the cells.

STRESS

It is not at all clear if stress causes tinnitus. What is clear is that stress is an inevitable part of our lives and is unavoidable. Lots of things can cause stress. Whether a prolonged period of stress or a stressful event, the resulting stress can make your tinnitus worse. It can often be a trigger that starts a vicious cycle of increased awareness of tinnitus leading to increased stress and therefore even more focus on the tinnitus.

EAR INFECTIONS

Some middle ear infections can cause tinnitus as well as a hearing loss. The resulting symptoms are generally temporary. It is important that any underlying infection is treated by a doctor though.

Ear Wax

Ear wax is by nature a waxy substance produced by the ear to clean and lubricate the ear canal. Although ear wax does not always cause a problem, excessive amounts produced in the ear canal can. Too much wax in the ear canal can cause a temporary hearing loss, pain as well as tinnitus.

Certain Medications

It is reported that there are about 200 medications that are known to cause tinnitus when you start or stop taking them. It must be stated that do not start taking or stop taking any medication without the consent of your doctor. Tinnitus is so variable from person to person that a medication might give someone the side effect of tinnitus whilst the same medication has no side effects on someone else. If you do experience tinnitus due to taking any medication, talk to your doctor about it if it is a concern.

The Noisy Body

It must be borne in mind that the body does not function in complete silence. There are many systems at work to keep you functioning and alive. These systems involve organs and arteries that are located near to the ears. It is not unusual to hear your respiratory system, movements of muscles as well as the sound of flowing blood. All can give rise to tinnitus.

FOOD AND DRINK

Although food and drinks do not cause tinnitus, some people have reported them exacerbating their tinnitus

The most common ones are; Caffeine, Alcohol, Tobacco, Salt, Spicy foods and Citrus fruits such as oranges.

Chapter 4. How The Ear Works

In understanding about tinnitus it is good to have a basic understanding of how the ear works and the hearing pathway.

The human ear is divided into three sections: the outer ear, the middle ear and the inner ear.

The Outer Ear

The outer ear is involved in the whole process of transmitting sound through to the middle and inner ears to be interpreted by the brain. The pinna which is a cup shaped device collects the sound from all directions. The amplified sound is then transmitted down the ear canal to the tympanic membrane or ear drum. The sound pressure wave then vibrates the ear drum.

The Middle Ear

The ear drum detects the vibration of sound and transmits it mechanically along a chain of three bones called the ossicles. The ossicles are made up of the malleus, the incus and the stapes. The malleus is attached to the inside part of the ear drum as well as to the incus. The incus is attached to the stapes. The stapes is attached to the oval window of the inner ear. The mechanical transmission of sound is converted into a sound pressure wave as the stapes acts like a small piston and pushes against the membrane of the oval window of the inner ear.

THE INNER EAR

The vibration of the oval window by the stapes footplate, sets in motion the sound pressure wave. The movement of the fluid is instantaneous throughout. This movement causes the basilar membrane to rise and fall to the same frequency and intensity of the incoming signal.

As the basilar membrane rises, so does the the organ of corti. The organ of corti contains the inner and outer hair cells and thus as the basilar membrane rises the hairs become displaced by the resistance from the overlying tectorial membrane. As the hairs become displaced there is a movement of ions from the positively charged endolymph (cochlea fluid) into the negatively charged hair cell.

This activity is the start of the neural signal, the sound pressure being transformed into electrical or neural activity. The greater the intensity of the incoming sound, the greater will be the displacement of hair cells. The greater the displacement, the greater the signal getting to the brain via the nerve pathway will be.

The Hearing Pathway

It is worth noting that it has been discovered that the hearing pathway has a complex filtering system. Although it is not fully understood yet, it does appear that the filtering system allows you to "zoom in" or "screen out" certain sounds that are of personal importance. The system works constantly to prevent you from being overwhelmed by your sound environment. The brain also has a response system which dictates how you react to certain sounds. These systems work closely together to control how you manage your sound environment. A good example of this is the "cocktail party scenario". Even if you might be engaged in a conversation with a group of friends, if you hear your name, you will try to "zoom in" on what is being said because it is important information about you.

You first hear your tinnitus because of the function of the hearing pathway, the filtering system and the sound response system. The tinnitus signal is first detected anywhere along the hearing pathway, commonly in the inner ear or on the auditory nerve. It can be so weak that it is sometimes not even detectable. However, if you do become aware of its presence, it will be because of the activity of your filtering system. How you respond to the tinnitus becomes crucial at this point because if you start to become stressed, annoyed and worried by it, those sound response systems will start to focus on it more. You will then hear it more and more.

There is some good news! These same sound and filter systems can be trained to ignore the tinnitus signals altogether. This process is called habituation and you know what that means – things will get better.

There have been studies carried out that show that with time and practice, the noises disappear completely or at the least reach a tolerable level in most cases, as the brain stops focusing on the signal. The length of time does vary from person to person but the main point is that it does happen.

There are various schools of thought and methods about how to go about treating tinnitus.

Chapter 5. Common Tinnitus Treatments

This chapter will explore some of the main methods of tinnitus treatments that involves habituation therapy.

INFORMATION

This may seem obvious but it can be missed. The more you know and educate yourself about tinnitus, the better you will begin to feel. You will soon discover that it is in fact extremely common and that you do not have to deal with it by yourself. You will have a sense of taking control of your tinnitus and getting your life back.

RELAXATION AND EXERCISE THERAPY

Learning to relax is probably one of the most effective ways to help with your tinnitus.

A lot of people with tinnitus find that the most exacerbating factor for tinnitus is stress. Tinnitus not only activates the auditory centre in the brain but also the emotional control centre, releasing stress hormones.

The impact of this is that the person becomes more stressed due to the tinnitus and this in turn increases the perception of the tinnitus even more.

Many people use music for relaxation and stress relief without even giving it a second thought. By selecting the right kind of appropriate music, a relaxed state can be achieved. The result is the breaking of the cycle of tinnitus and stress. More about this later on. But for now, let us consider other relaxation techniques.

The people who regularly practice relaxation techniques have stated that they reduce the overall loudness and intrusion of their tinnitus. They also become more indifferent to the tinnitus as well.

Some examples of relaxation techniques include deep breathing and progressive muscle relaxation. Some people find that taking part in activities such as Tai Chi and Yoga have proved to be beneficial as well.

Below is an example of a Deep Breathing exercise. This is the simplest of the relaxation procedures. It simply requires you to follow the instructions on deep, rhythmic breathing. Perform the exercise while sitting in a comfortable chair in a quiet place with no distractions; Remove your shoes and wear loose, comfortable clothing; Don't worry if you fall asleep; After finishing the exercise, close your eyes, relax for a few minutes, breathe deeply and rise up slowly.

Specifically, you should complete the following cycle 20 times:

 Exhale completely through your mouth; Inhale through your nose for four seconds (count "one thousand one, one thousand two, one thousand three, one thousand four"); Hold your breath for seven seconds; Exhale through your mouth for eight seconds; Repeat the cycle 20 times.

The entire process will take approximately 7 minutes.

SOUND THERAPY

Most people who experience tinnitus do so when it is quiet. Sound therapy, also known as sound enrichment, is when the quiet background is filled with therapeutic sounds. It is these sounds that act as a distraction from the tinnitus. By listening to some environmental or natural sound from a CD, a sound generator or even a fan, can help the brain to lessen and even ignore the tinnitus.

Some examples of sound therapy equipment include tinnitus relaxers and sound pillows.

COUNSELLING

This is extremely important when managing your tinnitus because it helps you to keep things in perspective and move forward in your learning to manage and habituate your tinnitus. Talking about your tinnitus and sharing how you feel about it can help you realise that you do not have to deal with tinnitus by yourself.

Two of the most common counseling treatments are Tinnitus Retraining Therapy and Cognitive Behavioural Therapy.

Tinnitus Retraining Therapy is a treatment which involves using a combination of sound therapy and directive counselling by a trained clinician. After an initial assessment a management plan is used to help the patient to habituate to their tinnitus.

Cognitive Behavioural Therapy basically involves changing the way you think about your tinnitus and your response behavior towards it. By dealing with the reasons that cause you distress, you are able to tolerate the consequences of your tinnitus more.

COMPLEMENTARY THERAPIES

There is a lot of information about these therapies around and to explore each one in depth is a book in itself. It does need to be kept in mind though, that these therapies do not treat the tinnitus but offer the patient a path to having a sense of wellbeing. This sense of relaxation and calm can help to deal with the stress associated with tinnitus. It is important that you realize that there has never been any conclusive evidence produced to show that any of these therapies work. If you want to try a particular therapy, do let your Doctor know.

Chapter 6. The Best Treatment For Tinnitus - For People With A Hearing Loss

If you ask any hearing aid audiologist about what they would consider to be the best treatment for tinntus, more often that not they will tell you that hearing aids are. I have experienced this for myself in the clinic that I run. I have been able to successfully treat patients who had tinnitus as well as a hearing loss with hearing aids.

Put it this way - Tinnitus patients feel better with hearing aids.

According to a survey among 230 hearing aid audiologists, the results showed that six out of 10 patients, that is 60%, experienced minor to major relief of tinnitus when wearing hearing aids. The survey also revealed that a total of one in five, that is 22%, received major relief.

Only less than 2% of patients experienced their tinnitus got worse, when wearing hearing aids, while 39% receive no benefit. Source: www.hearingreview.com

It has been observed that nearly everyone who has tinnitus also has some form of hearing loss.

Obviously, hearing aids should improve the hearing and communication of the patient. Unfortunately, what is not appreciated is the fact that hearing aids can also improve the tinnitus.

Firstly, there is a reduction in stress.

Without a hearing aid system people find communicating to be extremely stressful and hard work. When they start to use hearing aids, they increase their ability to communicate.

This in turn, reduces their stress level, and leaves them feeling better able to cope with their tinnitus.

Secondly, hearing aids provide a sort of sound therapy.

When a hearing aid system amplifies the background noise, the perception of the tinnitus is that it becomes less prominent

With the introduction of Open-fit hearing aids, it has been shown that these effects are even greater. In my experience of fitting Open-fit hearing aids, the results have been life changing for patients, whether NHS or private.

One manufacturer, called Widex, has taken this a step further and has incorporated programs within the hearing aids of specific types of music. They call them "Zen tones". The Zen tones are generated based on an understanding of the optimal music characteristics for relaxation.

One patient of mine had been living with raging tinnitus for some 40 years before he came to me for help. After being fitted with an appropriate Widex hearing aid system (including Zen tones), his wife told me it was like the hearing aid system had performed a miracle!

Chapter 7. The Best Treatment For Tinnitus - For People Without A Hearing Loss

Obviously, the last chapter is all well and good if you have a hearing loss. But what can be done for people who have tinnitus but have no hearing loss at all?

Well, Widex have come up with the solution to that problem as well.

The product is called Zen2Go.

According to Widex, the Zen2Go is efficient and demonstrates proven relief from tinnitus

So just exactly how does it work? The Zen2Go tinnitus management device plays random, soothing harmonic tones called Zen.

By using special tinnitus management technology, also known as fractal technology, combined with the latest hearing aid innovation, the Zen2Go device delivers you more sound, more words, a more natural listening experience and the opportunity to get relief from tinnitus.

The device sits behind the ear with a receiver being placed in the ear canal. It is light and comfortable and the wearer is not even aware of its presence.

Once placed in the ear, it is designed to help you relax and reduce stress – both of which help with tinnitus. Think of it as a relaxing, musical "spa" for your ears.

ZEN2GO comes in one box that contains everything you need

- A pair of ZEN2GO devices

- A matched RC-DEX

- User instructions forZEN2GO and RC-DEX

- Cleaning tools and extra ear-tips

Zen2Go is for all tinnitus sufferers. Plus, it has the benefit of being able to be worn immediately. No special fitting is needed. It is an added benefit if you can get the help of some counselling a professional though.

So, with this device combined with counselling from an experienced hearing aid audiologist trained in managing tinnitus, you can finally take control of your tinnitus.

CHAPTER 8. SPECIAL OFFER

I hope that you have found this guide useful. I want to encourage you to take control of your tinnitus and see an improvement in your quality of life. As a thank you for reading this guide, I want to make you a very special limited offer.

A Fantastic 30% Off

The High Street Price

Normally £1250.00 Each

Applies To Each

Zen2Go

Contact http://www.cshaa.co.uk

With This Coupon Code ZEN1*

*Terms and Conditions apply

1. Only one voucher per person.

2. You must use and quote the Coupon Code ZEN1.

3. This offer is subject to change at any time.

ABOUT THE AUTHOR

My name is Chris Scire, and for the past 10 years I have been a professionally qualified registered hearing aid audiologist. This includes being a Fellow of the British Society of Hearing Aid Audiologists and registered with the Health Care Professions Council. Over those years I have built up a good reputation within the industry. I was very successful as a branch manager with a national company before setting up my own practice. I was a finalist in the "Audiologist Of The Year 2012" competition out of over 500 UK audiologists.

I have met many people from all walks of life over the years and have experience in dealing with people's problems and frustrations. My philosophy is patient centred dispensing. This is carried out in a friendly personal consultative style, where nothing is too much trouble. I want you to have complete peace of mind when buying from my company. I have very competitively priced hearing aid solutions for you. I back this up with my no quibble 60 day money back guarantee and free aftercare for the life of the hearing aids. I don't use sales tactics to sell you the most expensive hearing aids.

If you have a question or just want a friendly chat, just contact me. chris@cshaa.co.uk I look forward to hearing from you.

Kind regards

Chris

Rev Chris Sciré BA PGCE DIPTH RHAD FSHAA

OTHER BOOKS BY YOUR NAME

Hearing Aid Prices Guide 2014

In the UK   https://tinyurl.com/ukedition

In the US   https://tinyurl.com/usaedition

Hearing Aids : How To Successfully Wear Hearing Aids

In the UK   https://tinyurl.com/ukedition

In the US   https://tinyurl.com/usaedition

ONE LAST THING... .

If you enjoyed this book or found it useful I'd be very grateful if you'd post a short review on Amazon. Your support really does make a difference and I read all the reviews personally so I can get your feedback and make this book even better.

If you'd like to leave a review then all you need to do is visit the book's review page on Amazon.

UK http://tinyurl.com/tinnitusuk

US http://tinyurl.com/tinnitususa

Thanks again for your support!

Tinnitus

DISCLAIMER

THE END